ZOLE 103

The Complete Mebendazole guide for treating parasitic worm infestations such as pinworm infections,roundworm infections,hook worm infections and whip worm infections effectively

Neta   Wilson

TABLE OF CONTENTS

THE MOST COMMON SIDE

CHAPTER 1

WHAT IS IT AND HOW DOES IT WORK

Infections caused by pinworms
(Enteroblus vermicularis),
roundworms (Ascaris
lumbricoides), whipworms
(Trichuris trichiura), and
hookworms (Ancylostoma
duodenale, Necator americanus)
can be treated with the medicine
mebendazole, which is available
only with a doctor's prescription.
Mebendazole is an anti-worm
medication that is effective
against a variety of worm
infestations. Anthelmintics are
the general name for this
category of drug, which includes

benbendazole. It achieves its effect by slaying the worms. It is an antiparasitic medication that is a member of the benzimidazole class, which is also comprised of the drugs thiabendazole, albendazole, and triclabendazole. In the same way as other benzimidazoles do, mebendazole eliminates parasites by preventing glucose uptake and disrupting the function of tubulin, which is an essential protein in parasites.

Emverm and Vermox are two different brand names that can be used to purchase mebendazole.

CHAPTER 2

BEFORE YOU TAKE MEBENDAZOLE, THESE ARE THE THINGS YOU SHOULD KNOW ABOUT ITS WARNINGS AND PRECAUTIONS

Geriatric

There is no information that can be found regarding the relationship between age and the effects that mebendazole has on individuals who are elderly.

Breastfeeding
There have not been any suitable studies conducted on women to determine whether or not using

this drug during breastfeeding poses a harm to the infant. Before taking any drug while nursing, make sure that you have the potential advantages weighed against the potential hazards.

Interactions Between Drugs

In some instances, it is OK to combine two distinct medications, even if there is a possibility that they will have an adverse interaction with one another. This is not the case for all medications, however. In certain circumstances, your physician may decide to adjust the dosage, or other preventative measures may be required. It is especially crucial that you let your doctor know if you are taking any of the other medications that are listed below if you are going to be taking this medication while you are also taking any of the other medications that are listed below. The following exchanges have been chosen because of the potential relevance they have; nonetheless, it should not be assumed that this list is exhaustive in any way.

Combining any of the following medications with this medication is not typically advised, but it is possible that doing so will be necessary in some circumstances. If your doctor prescribes both medications at the same time, he or she may adjust the dose or the frequency with which you take

either one or both of the
medications.

Other Interactions That Can Occur With Metronidazole

Certain drugs should not be taken
during, right before, or right after
eating meals or consuming
specific types of food due to the
likelihood of drug interactions.
Consuming alcohol or smoking
while taking certain medications
might further increase the risk of
an interaction occurring.Have a
discussion with the medical
professional who is treating you
regarding taking your medication
with food, drink, or tobacco.

Other Concerns Relating to Health

It is possible that the use of this medication will be impacted by the existence of other medical conditions. If you have any other medical issues, including but not limited to the following, be sure to inform your doctor.

If you have difficulties with your bone marrow, such as agranulocytosis or neutropenia, use this medication with extreme caution. May cause these symptoms to become even more severe.

Diseases of the liver: Use with extreme caution. May raise the likelihood of experiencing more severe adverse effects.

CHAPTER 3

CHOOSING THE APPROPRIATE DOSE AND METHOD OF ADMINISTRATION

Always make sure to adhere to the directions on the medication's label. Do not use this medication in greater or smaller doses than indicated, nor for a longer period of time than specified.

When treating whipworm, roundworm, and hookworm, the drug is often administered twice daily, once in the morning and once in the evening, for a total of three days. It is often administered as a single (one-time) dose in the course of treating pinworm. A single dose of the medication is normally given to the patient. If you are unable to chew the pill, place it on a spoon, and using a dosing syringe, administer a tiny amount of water onto the tablet. The amount should be between 2 and 3 milliliters. After two minutes, the tablet will have dissolved into a softer mass due to its absorption of the water and should then be ingested.

The initial dose consists of 100 milligrams taken twice daily for the first three days in order to treat specific infections caused by hookworms, roundworms, tapeworms, and whipworms. It is possible to take a mebendazole pill by mouth, to chew it, or to crumble it and mix it with food.

Take this medication for the full amount of time that is recommended by your doctor. Your symptoms could become better before the virus is completely gone. Skipping doses can also raise the likelihood that you will develop a secondary infection that is resistant to the antibiotics you are taking. A viral infection, such as the flu or the common cold, cannot be cured by the antibiotic mebendazole.

It is possible that you will need to continue taking this medication for anywhere from one to three days, depending on the disease that you are trying to treat. On the other hand, it can take up to three weeks before the infection is entirely cured.

Always be sure to wash your hands, including under your fingernails, but it's especially important to do so before eating and after using the restroom.

If the infection does not clear up during the first three weeks of treatment, you may require additional care.

In order to avoid being infected again, it is important to properly wash all of your clothes, linens, and towels and to do a thorough job of cleaning your home as directed by your physician. It's possible that other people in your household, including members of your family or other guests, will also need to take mebendazole or another medication. Infections caused by pinworms are very contagious and can transfer from one person to another.

It is not possible to get rid of a worm infestation by fasting (starving yourself), using laxatives, or making yourself throw up against your will. Take this medication exactly as advised for the greatest possible outcomes.
Missed dose:

If you are supposed to take mebendazole twice daily and you forget to take one of the doses, you should take the dose as soon as you remember it. If you remember more than four hours after the time that your dose was supposed to be taken, you should omit the missed dose and continue with your regular schedule. To compensate for a missing portion, don't take a twofold portion. Mebendazole overdose: It is highly improbable that taking an additional dose of this medication will harm you. You may, on the other hand, suffer from unpleasant side effects such as cramping in the stomach, feeling unwell, nausea, vomiting, and diarrhea. An unintentional overdose of a substance is a possibility. If you have taken more than the recommended amount of tablets, there is a possibility that you will have adverse effects on the functions of your body.

CHAPTER 4

THE MOST COMMON SIDE EFFECTS OF IT

The following are some of the more common adverse effects of benbendazole:

a rash, as well as nausea, vomiting, loss of appetite, diarrhea, and abdominal pain and discomfort.
Mebendazole can cause certain serious adverse effects, including the following:

symptoms such as hives, trouble breathing, swelling of the face, lips, tongue, or throat, sudden weakness, a sick feeling, fever, chills, sore throat, mouth sores, red or swollen gums, difficulty swallowing, easy bruising or bleeding, sores around the eyes, nose, mouth, or genital areas, and skin rash that spreads and causes blistering and peeling. Mebendazole may occasionally cause the following uncommon

Adverse effects:

CHAPTER 5

FAQ ABOUT IT

* Is Mebendazole safe?

When used in the amounts that your doctor recommends, mebendazole is one of the most effective antiparasitic medications available. It is also one of the safest. If you want to see favorable outcomes, you shouldn't stop taking Mebendazole too early without finishing the whole course of medication. Otherwise, your symptoms may come back or get worse. Mebendazole is risk-free when used in accordance with the recommended safety measures to prevent adverse reactions.

* How long does it take for the effects of benbendazole to wear off?

When mebendazole is taken orally, the bulk of the medication is absorbed into the gastrointestinal tract, where it continues to exert its antihelmintic activity locally. It stays in an active state and has a half-life that can range anywhere from three to six hours. When Mebendazole is administered orally, less than 2% of the medicine is removed in the urine, with the remaining 98% being excreted in the intestines as either unchanged pharmaceuticals or metabolites.

* Does Mebendazole kill all worms?

Mebendazole is used to treat only parasitic worm infections and anthelmintic gastrointestinal illnesses caused by Necator americanus (hookworm), Ancylostoma duodenale (hookworm), Ascaris lumbricoides (roundworm), Enterobius vermicularis (pinworm), and Trichuris trichiura (whipworm).

* What is the recommended dosage of Mebendazole?

Mebendazole may be administered as a single dose or as two separate doses, once daily for three days, depending on the kind of worm infection that the patient has. Your physician will provide you with instructions regarding the dosage and frequency of its administration. In addition, a follow-up treatment may be performed in a few weeks if it is deemed necessary to do so. In the case of other types of infections, heed

your physician's
recommendations.

* In which class of medications
does mebendazole fall?

Anthelmintics are a class of
medications that include
benbenazole, which is chemically
classified as a benzimidazole
carbamate. Mebendazole is under
the pharmacological category of
benzimidazole, and its
therapeutic application falls
under the category of
anthelmintic action.

* Does Mebendazole require a
prescription?

Mebendazole is a medicine that is used to treat parasites and worms. It is considered to be an antiparasitic. Even though it may be purchased without a prescription from stores that sell over-the-counter medicines, it is recommended that people only use it when under the care of a medical professional.

* Can Mebendazole cause liver damage?

When benbendazole is administered orally, it undergoes significant metabolism, the majority of which occurs in the liver. Plasma concentrations of its principal metabolites are significantly higher than those of benbendazole. Only in the presence of impaired hepatic function, metabolism, or biliary clearance, which can lead to elevated plasma concentrations of benbendazole, can it cause damage to the liver.

* Which is better, Albendazole or Mebendazole?

Both albendazole and mebendazole have a 100% success record in curing parasitic worm infections, making them exceptionally useful medications for treating the condition. For the treatment of several cases of Ascaris, hookworm, and Trichuris infections in large numbers, the benzimidazole derivative albendazole is the drug of choice.

THE   END

Printed in Great Britain
by Amazon